Copyright © 2009 Sandeep Grewal, M.D.

No part of this book may be copied, transmitted or republished in any form.

SECTION I
Basics of Physician Job Search

1. Physician Job Hunting Time line................................1
2. Getting Your Job Application Ready 9
3. Tips on Writing a Cover Letter.............................11
4. Where to Look For Physician Jobs.........................15
5. Physician Recruiters: *Whose Side Are They On?*......................*19*
6. The Physician Job Interview Process 25
7. What do the Physician Employers Want?.............................27
8. The Telephone Interview 29
9. The Interview Dress Code....................................33
10. The Rendezvous: *Anatomy of Physician Job Interview*.........*35*
11. In The Restaurant With Prospective Physician Employers....39
12. How to Evaluate a Job Opportunity like a Businessman 41
13. Physician Employment Contract 45
14. Physician Employment Benefits............................49
15. Should I Get My Physician Contract Reviewed? 53
16. Contract Negotiations 55
17. Getting Ready for Your First Physician Job 59
18. Are You Late for Physician Job hunt? *Last Minute Strategies .63*

SECTION II
Sample Questions: Physician Job Interview.................*65*

19. Sample Questions: *Private Practice Job Interview*..................*67*
20. Sample Questions: *Academic Medicine Job Interview*............*73*
21. Sample Illegal Questions and How to Answer them............77

DEDICATION

In the memory of my late Grandfather Mr. Jagir S. Grewal for his gift of education to everybody around him.

In the memory of my late Grandfather Mr. Harjit S. Bhangu for his effort to keep ancient medical remedies alive and passing them to the new generation.

PREFACE

We all learn a lot of new skills in medical school and residency. But when I came out of residency, I was unprepared for the business aspect of medicine. Contracts, interviews and even personal finance are somethings I learnt over a period of five years. Some by making mistakes myself, but mostly by observing others.

The most frustrating part is to see the same mistakes being made by young physicians over and over again. The mistakes are the same, only the faces change every year. I blame it on the lack of business training given to physicians. So I decided to write this book on physician job search, to answer questions which all medical residents and young physicians face at the beginning of their career as practicing physician.

The book is short and concise. It is a mini-guide. I never believed in long discharge summaries or lengthy prose. No physician or resident has time to devote days to a book. Therefore this mini-guide is to the point with no beating around the bush. It is short enough for you to be able to complete reading it in few hours. Both medical residents and young physicians in practice will find a gold mine of information relating to physician job search in this book.

For those who are wondering what is CareerMedicine.com all about. Here is the answer. CareerMedicine.com is my blog which is a platform to promote teaching business of medicine to residents and medical students. So when they graduate, they are not only excellent clinicians but also smart businessmen and women.

Cheers to all physicians who have struggled and established themselves in the harsh world of business without compromising their ethics.

Sandeep S Grewal, MD

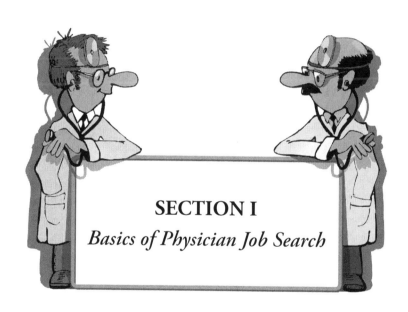

SECTION I
Basics of Physician Job Search

CHAPTER 1
Physician Job Hunting Time line

INTRODUCTION

What is the right time to start a physician job search? This question haunts every final year medical resident. There is one myth that needs to be clarified. Most of us are not sure how long the physician employers will wait for us to join the medical practice. This is the most common deterrent for the physicians to apply early. The truth is that most of the physician employers start anticipating need for a physician job opening many months and sometimes even a year or two in advance. Recruiting a physician is not easy. It takes several months of running advertisements, another four to six months to interview, couple of months to finalize the physician employment contract and so on. Even after accomplishing this entire task, employer has to wait many more months to complete credentialing and licensing for the incoming physician. Therefore employers like to finalize physician contracts as early as possible, even as early as one year, to give them enough time to complete all the formalities before actual start date. This pressure on the physician employer also makes it less likely for them to drop you if you are unable to join in time for some reason.

There are exceptions to the above mentioned time line especially when the need for a physician employee is acute. Acute need arises in cases such as a physician abruptly leaving the practice or sudden increase in patient volume. Even these employers may be forced to wait; if they are not able to find someone to start immediately.

Meanwhile they fill up the position temporarily with locum tenens till the new physician is able to begin the employment.

THE PREPARATION

Unfortunately you cannot jump out of the bed one fine morning and start looking for the physician job. Just as physician employers have to plan months and even a couple of year in advance to announce a vacancy, you have to start planning your physician job search too. There are several variables. Do you want to go for a job or you want to do a fellowship? Do you want to go solo, join a group practice or become a partner? Do you want to be an academician or go into a private practice? What states do you want to consider a job opportunity in? And the list goes on.

You may also want to talk to people who are already doing what you want to do. They may be able to tell you pros and cons and may even lead to a change of heart. Or vice versa, make you even more determined to get the same kind of job.

Once you have decided the type of job you will be applying to, you will need to prepare a resume and cover letter to promote your strong points. You may need to acquire extra skills, put in extra time to do research or learn procedures so that you can outshine other candidates.

THE HUNT

Now when you are ready with your ammunition to succeed in the battle of finding the right job, there is more to do. You need to fish out opportunities. Many good physician employment opportunities in medicine are not advertised and are filled by word of mouth. This is why networking is important. You will need to scour listings in the classifieds of various journals, call them to find more about the physician job opportunity and then fax or email your resume. Then you will need to follow up on the applications. It gets challenging to juggle your time between your present responsibilities, upcoming board exams etc. with your physician job search. That again gives me an opportunity to emphasize the importance of getting a running start, early in the game.

By the beginning of the final year of your residency program, you should have had it all thought out. What field you are going to pursue, where will you settle down, and what you should add to your skills to make yourself marketable. Beginning of the final year of your residency should be about resume writing and finalizing your application. Also cover letters should be drafted. Make standard cover letters for different fields you plan to apply to. Keep back up copies on your computer, on a disc, as well on the web. So you can access them whenever you want to. You can keep your resume and cover letter saved as attachments in your email. This way they will be available to you on the go.

The aim is to sign a physician employment contract within the first six months of your final year. You will need rest of the year to complete your credentialing and other paperwork. That leaves you with six months to complete your mammoth task of physician job hunting. I have developed a time line, on the next page, that you can refer to. Make sure you complete all the work in a given month so that you don't lose the acceleration you have gained by starting early.

RECOMMENDED CALENDAR FOR JOB SEARCH:

End of Second Year or Preferably at the Beginning of Your Residency

- File application with Federation of Credential Verification Service to get your credentials verified. This will make your future license applications much quicker. I would especially recommend it if you are a foreign medical graduate. It will eliminate the need to get your credentials verified by your medical school again and again.

You can get an application form from 1-888-ASK-FCVS *or online at* www.fsmb.org

JULY
- Write your cover letters (*one week*)
- Finalize your resume (*one week*)
- Decide your priorities in looking for a job (*one week*)
- Show your resume and cover letter to peers and mentors for corrections and suggestions
- Decide what month you will be interviewing and schedule an easy rotation or vacation for yourself

AUGUST
- Start scouring journals/ websites for physician job classifieds and make an excel sheet to list them
- Enroll with physician recruiters
- Talk to your mentors regarding the job you want and see if they know about an opening.
- Get a fax machine at home/ work secured for your use.
- Start faxing or emailing your resume to prospective physician employers.

SEPTEMBER

- Continue looking for physician employment opportunities in various medical journals
- Continue faxing your resume/ cover letter
- Start calling prospective physician employers one week after sending your resume.
- Schedule interviews for the month you have selected.

OCTOBER

- Continue what you did in September
- Attend interviews

NOVEMBER

- Continue attending interviews.
- Continue job search if you are not pleased with the places where you are getting interviews from.
- Decide by end of the month where you will join.
- Make sure you have registered for the medical boards.
- Register for a board review course in your specialty.

DECEMBER

- Reply to your prospective physician employer about your decision to join the group.
- Obtain the physician employment contract
- Get the physician contract reviewed by an attorney
- Negotiate the contract
- Sign the physician employment contract

JANUARY

- Apply for state medical license
- Apply for hospital privileges (*even if license pending*)
- Fill and send employment paperwork
- Fill and send credentialing paperwork for medical insurance companies, HMOs etc.(*Payors*)

FEBRUARY
- Call and find out if your employer has everything they need
- Try to find out about housing in the area
  you will be moving to.
- CAUTION: Don't buy a house until you are at least six
  months into the job.

MARCH
- ENJOY!…..AH! *well…study for the boards.*

APRIL
- STUDY HARDER!

MAY
- EVEN HARDER!!

JUNE
- Plan your moving out
- Arrange for an apartment or a house near your work area.
- Reserve the movers well in advance.
- Make sure you attend your graduation party. You will not
  get another chance.
- Attend a board review course

JULY
- Get Back to Work. ■■■

CHAPTER 2
Getting Your Job Application Ready

Fortunately the application process to apply for a physician job is very simple. All you need is a cover letter and a resume or curriculum vitae. There is no need to send your credentials, certificates or other documents at the time of application. Some employers, especially academic institutions will ask for names and addresses of your references. Very rarely they may request actual recommendation letters. That is unusual.

You can send your application by mail, fax or even email. While sending email documents always send them as attachments in .rtf format instead of .doc. It is also called the 'rich text format' (.rtf) and enables the recipient to open the document in almost any edition of Microsoft Word or even Notepad. Try not to use your Macintosh Computer as most institutions and offices still use IBM. Documents generated in a Mac may not look good on a PC.

Always email your application packet to yourself or a friend to see if there is any problem with the format of the resume or letter. Such errors can look ugly showing up on the recipient side as line displacements, change of fonts etc. Never ever skip this simple quality control step before sending your application to prospective employers. ■■■

CHAPTER 3
Tips on Writing a Cover Letter

Cover letter is a very important part of your physician employment application. Your application has only two papers in it, that is your cover letter and your resume or curriculum vitae. The prospective medical employer will read your cover letter first and then your resume.

Your cover letter should refer to kind of position you are looking for, your basic medical training, your strengths and the best way to reach you. Don't get long winded. No one has time to read a chapter. That is one reason I have kept this book short. If you are applying for more than one type of physician jobs then you need to make separate cover letters for each of them. Also as we realize that we are not applying to McDonalds, we should personalize the letter to each physician employer by adding the contact person's name into the letter. It's a lot of paper to print when you will be sending seventy to eighty applications but fortunately it is easier to do it with the help of computers.

Use the following tips to draft your cover letter and you should end up with a decent prose. You can also look at some sample cover letters from many other books on job search before you draft yours. The points are in the sequence in which you will be drafting your letter.

- Date the letter and change the date when necessary

- Give your current address including a cell phone number or beeper number so it is easier for your employers to contact you. Encourage them to leave message if you are not available

- Give your current email address

- Correctly spell the name of the contact person to whom you are sending the letter

- Never generalize your letter unless you have absolutely no information. Refer to your employer as Dear Mr. or Ms. or Dr. X as the case may be

- If you don't know who to address the letter to, then call and find out

- Keep the body of the letter short and sweet

- First paragraph should mention your medical specialty and institute of training. Also make a note about your board certification status i.e. whether you are board eligible or board certified. Write when you would be available to start your physician employment. Keep the first paragraph limited to three to four sentences.

- Second paragraph should highlight your strengths in the field. If you are applying to a private practice you can mention various procedural skills you possess. Remember knowledge of extra procedures gives you an edge to generate more revenue for the medical practice. Private practices love it!

- If you are going for the academics then blow the trumpet about your research experience and other academic achievements. Be creative and think what the physician employer may be looking for in a particular setting. But please! Keep it short. Not more than four lines. And No! You cannot use extra long sentences to get around it.

- Last paragraph is generally *"Looking forward to hear from you…. blah blah blah"*. But also use this space to inform the prospective physician employer about the best way to contact you. That is your email, cell or beeper number.

- Do not forget to put MD or DO behind your name

- Do sign your name

- Some books will suggest you to write a small sentence at the end by hand to give a personal touch to the letter. You may do it provided you have a decent handwriting. I guess that leaves ninety nine percent of us docs out. ∎∎∎

CHAPTER 4
Where to Look For Physician Jobs?

Where can you find physician jobs? They seem to be everywhere, yet when you call around there seem to be none. The reason for that is there are only one or two openings per institution unless it is a hospital or health care system. To add to the confusion, the good jobs somehow are never advertised as they are filled by word of mouth. So here are few ways you can search for them.

1 JOURNALS: Look in the classified sections of journals such as New England Journal of Medicine (NEJM) or Journal of American Medical Association (JAMA). These two journals carry recruitment advertisement for all specialities. Tip! It is easier to search the listing online at the websites of these journals.

2 SPECIALTY JOURNALS: Look in the classified section of your specialty journals. You will find a hidden source of listings there which may not be huge but more.

3 FACULTY: Check with the faculty of your residency program if they know of any of their contacts looking for a physician. They may have contacts all over the country and they always get enquiries on finding a good candidate.

4 PHYSICIANS AROUND YOU: Make sure every physician around you knows that you are looking for a job. Make the whole issue public. You never know who is the right person to talk to.

5 PHYSICIAN RECRUITERS: Many medical practices resort to physician recruiters as it is cumbersome to find a physician. This is a complicated matter so I have dedicated a full chapter to it.

6 DRUG REPS: Yes they would know. Since they go all around the town talking to physicians in various practices, they usually have an idea who is looking for a physician.

7 COLD CALL: If you are interested to get a job in a particular city or town, just call the medical practices there to see if they are looking for a physician. Try to talk to the practice manager or the physician in charge.

8 LOCUM TENENS: You can consider doing locum tenens for few months to find out a good opportunity. Usually the practices hiring locum tenens are using them because they do not have a permanent candidate. If they like your work and you like their job, then why not.

DIRECT MAIL:
An Innovative Way of Physician Job Search

Direct mail is a method used by business people and retailers to send unsolicited mail to potential customers. Marketing is not a random science. It is very systematic. If you send 10 resumes you will get 2 interviews. If you send out a 100, you will get 20 interviews. If you send out a thousand you will get 200 interviews!!! The ratio may be different for each specialty and each person but basics of marketing are the same.

So why not use this marketing method to find jobs. After all looking for a job is no less than marketing ourselves to the physician employer. So here is what you should do.

STEP 1: Find out a list of medical practices in your specialty in the location you are interested in. You can buy a list, you can search local yellow pages or you can look it up online.

STEP 2: Mail a resume and a cover letter to each of these practices or better still, each of the physicians in the practices.

If a physician or physician group is planning to hire in the near future, just getting your resume will save them a lot of money, time and headaches. Others may be tempted to add another physician to their practice. ∎∎∎

CHAPTER 5
Physician Recruiters: Whose Side Are They On?

Do you get hundreds of phone calls from various physician recruiters? Ever wondered whose side are they on? Let us find out.

Physician recruiters are salespeople. There job is to sell you a 'physician job' or a 'physician job interview' depending on how the recruiters get paid. There is big money to be made in physician recruiting (Sometimes double of the monthly salary offered for the physician job!).

The physician recruiters contract with physician employers and may elect to get paid if they are able to send a physician candidate for interview. Or they may instead elect to get a bigger payout only if a physician signs up for the job.

For a recruiter, who is getting paid just to get candidates into the door for physician interviews, his main objective will be to get as many interviews set up as possible. An unethical recruiter will not care whether the physician job suits you or not. He will not care whether the physician employer may like that candidate or not. He would want you to just show up for the interview. So if you get those kind of calls from recruiters, who are pushing you to go to a certain desolate place for an interview, that's what it is all about. If the recruiter gets paid only if a physician candidate signs up for the doctor job, they have to be more careful about selecting physician applicants to recommend for interviewing. But again, they would like to send more candidates in to increase the chances of filling the physician job.

Lets look at an example: The physician recruiter is an agent for two physician jobs: Job opening A and Job opening B. Job Opening A is a lucrative physician job in Beverly Hills and Job opening B is in the middle of Sonoran Desert. If the recruiter is supposed to get double commission for filling up the Sonoran Desert physician job opening, then its obvious he will try to sell that position first. If he comes across a medical resident who sticks to his job criteria, and refuses to go to middle of no where, not even for an interview, then the recruiter may disclose the position in Beverly Hills.

Summary: Physician recruiters are salesmen. They will try to nudge you to go for physicians jobs which offer them more commission. They probably care the least about what physician candidate wants or what physician employer wants. Hopefully you will bump into a good physician recruiter. But keep your guards up.

PHYSICIAN RECRUITERS:
How To Handle Them

There are various conflicts of interest involving the physician recruiters, the physician employer and the physician candidate. But you should not completely cut them out of your job search strategy. Physician recruiters many times do have access to some great opportunities. If you are able to partner with a good recruiter, job search can be slightly easier.

There are certain rules I used, when I had to deal with physician recruiters. It helped me avoid unnecessary interview trips, sidestep unwanted physician jobs and prevent pesky calls from them at work.

1 What do you want?

Develop the criteria of an ideal job. List the "must haves" and never ever deviate from them unless you are in dire straits.

2 'Call me' preferences

Let the physician recruiter know in the beginning when and how you would like to be contacted.

3 Push the pushy recruiter

If the recruiter is too pushy and comes onto you too strong, then dump him. If a physician recruiter is trying to dictate which job you should take or which interview you should go to, then he probably has a conflict of interest involved.

4 Don't please them, they should please you

Physician recruiters are like real estate agents. The are supposed to find the candidates for the physician jobs and a suitable job for you. Giving them too much say in deciding what you should do will not help. They cannot hire you. They can forward your application in the right or wrong direction.

5 They are not the only one

Do not forget other ways of physician job hunting. Do not depend on recruiters solely. Plus there are hundreds of recruiter agencies you can deal with.

6 Ask for a change

A physician recruitment company may have several agents. If you do believe that the company has a better job opening but your agent is not presenting them to you, then ask for a change. Ask to speak to their supervisor and request a change of agent. Otherwise no matter which way you try to approach the agency, you will end up with the same guy as "he is handling your case"

UNDERSTANDING PHYSICIAN RECRUITER ADVERTISEMENT

On a lighter note, here is the code for understanding those mailers sent to you by the Physician recruiters:

1 Located in the heart of paradise = *a very, very rural area*

2 Charm of a small town life = *Here fine-dining is the local Chinese buffet*

3 Easy access to all amenities = *If you drive couple of hours looking for it!*

4 15 minutes inland from the ocean = *Be careful! Lots of hurricanes!!*

5 For those who love outdoor activities = *It is deep in the jungle.*

6 Enjoy year long skiing = *You got it! Very very cold!!*

7 Opportunity of a lifetime = *We are having tough time finding applicants*

8 Opportunity to do it all = *No specialists available around... you will be on your own*

9 Low cost of living = *If you buy that house in the Ghettos*

10 Option of Partnership track = *Just kidding!!* ■■■

NOTES

Collect your physician recruiters contact information here for future reference

CHAPTER 6
The Physician Job Interview Process

INTRODUCTION

Hiring decisions in the world of medicine are not made without face-to-face interviews. Interviewing techniques for the academia and the private sector differ markedly. The expectations are different, the questions are different and the answers are different. What may sound offending or lame in academia may become the prime topic of discussion in a private setting. These are different perspectives in medicine and does not necessarily mean either one is bad.

[Apparently the academicians appear to have principles while private practitioners come across as businessmen. However do not forget that the academia gets most of its funding from federal and state programs or grants. Whereas the private practitioner has to generate his own capital to keep his practice viable. In reality all successful practitioners are good businessmen. As long as the practice of medicine is fair and ethical you have nothing to fear.]

THE PROCESS

The first contact with the prospective employer is by telephone. Usually the prospective employer initiates the call. At the end of this conversation you may or may not be offered an interview. Occasionally you may get a call from office personnel to schedule an interview.

The face-to face interviews are by and large unstructured interviews where your academic knowledge is almost never tested. Your graduation from medical school and completion of residency are sufficient proof of your academic competence. If everything goes well in the interview and your references check out well, you are likely to be offered the job in next few days to weeks. ■■■

CHAPTER 7
What do the Physician Employers Want?

As a candidate for a physician job, you make an assessment of an opportunity largely based on background research, compensation, location etc. most of which you know beforehand. The prospective employer makes a decision based on your performance in the interview. That's why these interviews are intimidating. But if you know what they are looking for, it will become much easier for you to sell yourself.

Prospective physician employees are generally evaluated against the following criteria, so be ready to demonstrate your ability in these areas:

1 Is the physician candidate qualified to do the job?

2 Does he or she have good communication skills?

3 Will he or she fit into our team?

4 Is the candidate interested to work with us?

5 Are their any red flags that may hinder procurement of medical licenses, malpractice insurance, credentials etc?

6 What is the advantage to the employer if we chose him or her over other physician candidates? ■■■

CHAPTER 8
The Telephone Interview

Going for a physician job interview is by itself a energy draining commitment. Before a face-to-face interview with the physician candidates, the prospective employers screen them over the phone. This is because interviewing involves a significant monetary and time commitment. Hence the physician employers need to know few important things about you beforehand. It is also to your advantage as you can ask specific questions regarding the physician job to determine if you want to attend the job interview or not. Expect each telephone interview to last anywhere from ten minutes to thirty minutes. If it is the recruiter calling you then you probably will be done much faster. Following are the few important issues the interviewer is digging into:

1 How did you hear about us?

It sounds easy, but it isn't so! Many a times when you get that unexpected call from the potential employer you would not even remember whether you found the physician job listed in NEJM, JAMA or online. Non-specific answers like "one of the journals" or "online" are acceptable but being specific may project a better image of yours. The answer to it is not as important by itself, as the question is generally used as an icebreaker. But if you came to know about the physician job by networking, do not forget to mention who referred the position to you. References in the medical field may work wonders.

2 Are you serious about this physician job and the interview process?

They won't ask you directly but you will have to make them feel that you are serious and interested in the job opening. After all physicians are busy with their practice, and even if you are paying for the job interview logistics, they would not like to waste their time interviewing you if you are not serious about the position at their facility.

3 Are you willing to relocate?

If they offer you the job would you be willing to move to the area? The employers realize that this is a very significant factor while considering job offers for doctors. They may try to make sure that your spouse or significant other is also into the relocation.

4 Can you hold a good conversation?

In medicine your ability to communicate reflects how you good are you with patient communication. Tip! To improve your performance in a phone job interview, record your voice on a tape and listen to it. You will find few things you may want to change.

The employers also use this opportunity to explain to you what the medical job entails. Most of the time the private physician employer will also tell you about the compensation package *(Salary and Benefits)*. After all they also have to attract you to their medical practice.

Typically you will not be able to attend more than 4 to 6 in person job interviews, hence you should also use this interaction to screen whether you want to attend this interview or not.

Questions you should ask:

1 Ask about the locality (Total population, nearest big city etc.) to get an idea where it is.

2 Make efforts to clarify anything that is vital for you to decide whether you want to take that position or not.***

3 If you are a foreign medical graduate confirm beforehand if they are willing to sponsor visa/immigration. Do not wait till you get there.

4 If the interview is from private sector you can ask them if they will reimburse your expenses for the interview before agreeing for one. If the call is from academia then leave the question for the office secretary who you can call later in the day.

*** *The best way to approach this would be to develop criteria to screen physician job interview offers. For example: Places with population more than 20,000, salary over $150,000, must offer medical insurance, should not be more than thirty minutes drive from a big city etc. Include everything that is vital for you. The factors that are negotiable for you can be used to rank these job interview offers in a preferential order. But be flexible. It is hard to find the ideal job. By and large you gain some and lose some points.* ■■■

CHAPTER 9
The Interview Dress Code
"To be successful, look successful"

Men: Conservative business suit (preferably two different ones for more than one day physician job interviews!). If you have only one suit then change your shirt and tie each day. You do not need to wear traditional navy blue or black suit with white shirt. Try something different, which brightens up your face. Lighter shades work good for people with dark skin and those who are slim. For those who are on the heavier side should buy darker shades. Buy you suit well in advance in anticipation and not in the last minute. This may save you money during sales of name brand suits and will give you enough time to find the one that you like. It is important that the suit you wear makes you feel confident about yourself, as it will show on your face.

Pay special attention to your shoes, ties, belts and watches. They should not look worn out. Shoes have to be brown or black depending upon the color of your suit and of course should be of same color as the belt. No perfumes please. Deodorant is a must but prefer the odorless ones. Your aftershave should not have a long lasting strong smell. Use a mild one.

Women: Women should also wear a conservative business suit. If you are wearing a skirt let it be at least below mid thigh. Wearing slacks instead is an acceptable alternative. And if a suit does not make you feel confident, it is not the right one for you either. Always wear stockings with skirts, which should be of natural color. No glitter on your stockings please. Again if you are not slim try wearing darker colors. Women should also consider having two sets of clothing for those more than two days interviews.

Keep jewelry to the minimum. Bling-bling is not acceptable. Do not wear a noticeably high heel. Take a briefcase or handbag instead of a purse. No perfumes for you too. Wear an odor-less deodorant. You may wear makeup but don't get heavy handed. Excessive make up will undermine your confident image. ■■■

CHAPTER 10
The Rendezvous
Anatomy of Physician Job Interview

To highlight this difference in approach regarding the physician job interview, discussions will be divided into two categories 'academia' and 'private'.

THE SCENARIO

Private: Most physician job interviews for private medical practice are conducted over one to two days, one day being more common. The job interview of physicians is generally informal. During the day you can expect tour of the group's medical office or offices and the hospital. The prospective physician employer tries to entice you with the grandeur and facilities of their working place. You can expect to be driven around the town in an effort to attract you to the area. Generally the spouse is also invited to the interview. Serious discussions take place at lunch or dinner in a good restaurant.

Academia: Interview for the academic physician job openings are more formal and conducted by multiple physician faculties either as a group or separately. These job interviews usually last one full day or two days at most. You will meet most of the senior physician faculty in their administrative offices and can expect questions similar to the one you answered during your residency program interviews. You will be given the tour of the institution but not of the locality. Lunch is usually provided during an informal session with other physician faculty giving you an opportunity to ask questions.

THE EXPECTATIONS

Private: Private medical groups are not searching for the brightest guy. If you have the required credentials to practice medicine and you are a good fit into their group it is more than enough. They are least concerned with your academic merits or research activities. They are looking for someone who can work hard and survive in the business; someone motivated to advance the group's dealings. If you are skillful at a generously paying medical procedure, consider yourself ahead of the game. They also want you to be flexible during unexpected staffing shortages. Being a team player is important.

Academia: Physician compensation in academic medicine is generally less than that offered by private sector. For this reason, they want to make sure you really want to be in academics by choice. Most of the questions would be directed towards this concern. Your academic merits, research projects, published articles and teaching experience matter the most here. Your ability to generate grants may become a serious concern for them especially if you are interviewing primarily for a research position. Also keep you list of references ready.

Unless you are a senior faculty already or are applying primarily for a research position, the percentage of time you want for devoted research activities will be an important issue they will consider. If you are interviewing for a clinical position and you are asking for a significant research time, consider yourself out.

THE FIRST IMPRESSION
"A bad impression is the last impression"

In any job interview the first impression may not be the last impression. But if you mess up somewhere, that will surely be a long lasting one. Interviews are like rock climbing. You may be doing quite well and you may be almost there. But make one mistake and you will slip all the way down to square one. Nevertheless first impression has enormous value. And here's how to make a good one.

- SMILE

- SMILE!

- SMILE!! *(Alright! not so profusely)*

- Eye contact *(intermittently without making it look like a stare!)*

- Firm handshake *(Neither a limp handshake nor a bone crushing one is good. And never use a two-hand handshake. We are not at a funeral of our hopes.)*

- Walk confidently.

- Don't forget the small talk. *(Don't forget to ask your interviewer also 'How are you?')*

- Be polite.

CLOSING

Always leave the physician job interview with a positive note. Do let the employer know that you certainly found the practice opportunity appealing and would definitely consider it strongly while making a decision. They may be keen to know how soon you will be able to make a decision, especially if they are interested in you. If you are offered the spot at the interview itself, do not get pressurized to accept it. In fact never accept it right away. You ought to go back to your room and think it over!

HOW DID YOU DO?

Well unless an job offer is made, it is very difficult to find out how you did. But certain cues are helpful in assessing your performance during the job interview.

If the prospective physician employer cancels the job interview midway for any reason, chances are that he does not want to waste anymore of his time interviewing you. Sorry!

If the medical employer thanks you and would let you know about his decision in a few weeks, then you did well but he wants to take a look at other candidates.

If the medical employer is wondering when you will be able to make a decision or if he promises you that you will hear from him in the next day or two, then you have nothing to worry about. You made your point. ■■■

CHAPTER 11
In The Restaurant With Prospective Physician Employers

Interviews for private practice openings including most of the discussions regarding salary, benefits, job requirements etc take place over a lunch or a dinner at an upscale restaurant. There is a tendency to lose ones guard in these informal setting. But don't!! Following are certain do's and don'ts during lunch/ Dinner interviews.

The Do's
- Be polite to everybody you meet *(including the waiters)*
- Make note of any point of importance
- Appear relaxed...But inside do not relax – keep your guard up!
- Do smile occasionally *(NOT always!)*
- Listen attentively
- Before leaving any office or location,
  discuss what the next step is *(If it is to visit someplace then take directions/ addresses very carefully)*
- Keep pager / cell phone in silent mode

The Don'ts
- Do not interrupt when someone else is speaking
- Do not order alcoholic beverages
- Do not order messy foods *(Soups and salads are good choices)*
- Do not order very expensive food
- Do not overeat

- Do not offer to pay
- Do not talk with a mouthful of seafood waiting to come out
- Do not take big bites
- Do not eat fast
- Do not smoke ■■■

CHAPTER 12
How to Evaluate a Physician Job Opportunity like a Businessman.

These are the pointers you cannot ignore when evaluating a physician job opportunity. It is not just gut feeling, but objective data that counts. The diligence you put in to evaluating the job opportunity, during and after the interview, will determine your job satisfaction in an year or two.

1. SALARY: That is a no brainer. You need higher salary to pay off your loans and to live comfortably as well as save for retirement.

Also make sure your time is adequately compensated. You are not supposed to do anything for free. Well not anymore! A friend of mine was offered a part-time position with hourly pay and then asked to cover night calls for free. The excuse was that the practice is new and until it builds up they cannot offer a full time position but someone has to take the call. If that ever happens to you remember you are not responsible for cutting cost for someone else's business ramp up period.

The only reason you should do it is for your own business or if you are already a physician partner. Unfortunately, there are many physician employers out there, who would love to have you sacrifice for their business without giving you a partnership deal. Remember if you are an employee, you charge like an employee. If you are a partner then you do whatever you can to help the medical practice. But don't be a hard-liner either. Once in a while if a need arises do pitch in because that projects you as a reliable person.

2. FINANCIAL STRENGTH: The medical practice you are about to join will usually guarantee you salary and benefits. If the company is not financially sound, it may not be able to keep the word and you may end up looking for another job very soon. This is especially critical for foreign medical graduates who plan to file their immigration application through the new employer, or for those with families to relocate.

Trying to find out financials of a company is nearly impossible but you can get an idea from the county website to see if the property taxes are being paid on time or not. You can also check with other doctors in the practice and see if they receive their pay checks, bonuses, reimbursement for CME's etc in time. You can also ask the question directly at the job interview. See if you get a wishy washy answer or a straightforward declaration of profitability.

You can talk to other physicians in the area and they may be able to give you some idea. But take it with a grain of salt as it may be nothing but some juicy gossip. Look for consistency. If the physician employer is in a financially bad position, they may tell you that how your addition to the practice will help them boost revenues and bring them out of red. However never become a passenger in a sinking ship. If physicians already there are losing money why would a new addition change it. Even the banks don't loan to a losing business, why should you?

3. PHYSICIAN TURNOVER: Be very careful if you hear these stories about physicians leaving the practice and new physicians entering all the time. A revolving door for employees means the corporation is not able to keep anyone happy. And if they cannot keep the physician there happy, there is no way they will keep you happy.

It is expensive to recruit a physician and the ramp up period to establish a physician is also costly. Therefore most medical groups try to retain physicians by trying to keep them happy. Those who can't, lose a lot of time , money and effort in the process and are usually declining financially.

4. PAYER MIX: You need to examine the payer mix in the area as it is directly linked to your revenues. The term is used to describe the percentage of Medicare, Medicaid, Private Insurance and Uninsured population in the area. Again I strongly believe that all patients should receive decent medical care irrespective of their insurance status. However payer mix will determine how many patients you will have to see a day to make your salary. Unfortunately payer mix has become very important in this era of Medicare cutbacks.

5. REPUTATION: Reputation of a practice, although ignored by many, is very important. Check with other physicians and consultants around the area to see if the group is reputable. If you join some infamous group, you will instantly become infamous. If you join a well respected group in town, you will get some of that respect even on the first day.

6. OFFICE DYNAMICS: Closely observe the way staff treats each other and their patients. Usually that reflects how the management treats the staff. And that is how you will be treated.

7. SUPPORTING SPECIALTY PHYSICIANS: Make sure you are comfortable with the kind of cases the practice deals with. If you are an Family Practitioner and don't want to deliver babies, don't join a group that does it. Or make it clear before you sign up. Put it in the contract. Make sure there are specialists around for you to refer a complex case to. ■■■

CHAPTER 13
Physician Employment Contract

Ah! At last the dotted line. Hopefully by now you have the physician employment contract in your hand. This section helps you understand a Physician Employment Contract (PEC) also called Physician Employment Agreement (PEA). Also there are some things you want or do not want in a contract. We will go over all of that in this chapter.

Remember to read the Physician Employment Contract yourself, at least three to four times before you even send it out to your attorney for review. You may not be able to understand it the first time but by the fourth reading you will definitely have some idea.

Some of the contracts are written in a simple language, but others may be more difficult than reading the unabridged Shakespeare play. In the following pages, I will list some of the things you need to watch out for in a physician employment contract. Remember, if it is not written, it is not agreed upon.

Anything included in this book is not a legal advice and you must consult your attorney prior to signing any contract. The information listed here is for informational purposes only.

Here are some of the essential components of an employment contract which you may find:

SALARY:
Your guaranteed salary should always be mentioned on the physician employment contract. Never ever sign a job contract without a written guaranteed salary (unless you don't want a guaranteed salary!).

BENEFITS:
Benefits are usually attached as an appendix to the contract.

VACATION:
Do make sure that vacation time is clearly written out on the contract. Sick leave and CME leave should also be listed separately or documented as included if that is the case.

EXIT STRATEGY:
Both parties should be able to get out of the contract without any reason. Usually it requires a three to six months notice. Thus neither you nor your employer is trapped in an undesirable situation.

TERMINATION WITH CAUSE:
"Nothing is guaranteed if you do anything wrong"
This section allows the employer to terminate your employment for any reason listed in this section. Make sure all these reasons are justifiable and do not give the employer a free hand in firing you.

TERMINATION WITHOUT CAUSE:
"Nothing is guaranteed if you do anything right"
This section allows both parties to terminate the contract after giving a usual three to six month notice.

RESTRICTIVE COVENANT:
If a physician employee leaves the practice, a restrictive covenant bars him for working in a predetermined area (usually 5 to 10 miles around the practice) for a limited period of time (one to two years usually).

RESPONSIBILITY:

Call schedule, weekend coverage, hospital coverage are to be divided equally among the physicians of same specialty. It should be written in the contract. A simple statement stating calls will be divided amongst the physicians in a practice is different than stating that calls will be divided EQUALLY.

EARNINGS FROM MOON LIGHTING, MEDICAL DIRECTORSHIP OR OTHER BUSINESS:

Many a times contracts will assign all your earnings from moonlighting, medical directorship etc to the company. That is not right. Your earnings from any other business except employment cannot be gobbled up like this. Make sure you them get to delete any such clause.

BONUS FORMULA:

You should be making bonus once your productivity reaches beyond a certain mark. Usually it is in dollar amount of revenue generated by you. Sometimes it may be a number of patients seen or other methods to calculate a physician's productivity. Whatever that formula is should be clearly written down in the contract. Do not accept verbal promises for bonuses.

PROFESSIONAL LIABILITY INSURANCE:

Employers have traditionally provided and paid for professional liability insurance for full time physician employees. That should be mentioned in the contract.

Try to avoid employers who do not pay for professional liability insurance. Even though it may be cheaper to obtain a liability insurance in your first few years of practice, it can go up significantly more as patients and years add to your medical practice. ■■■

CHAPTER 14
Physician Employment Benefits

Compensation as a physician employee consists of Salary plus Benefits. You need to know what benefits you can get before you begin negotiations. If the physician employer is not willing to raise the physician salary, you can ask for more benefits and add value to the compensation. Also the benefits can help you differentiate between two jobs offering the same physician salary.

Sometimes benefits offered have to be same for all employees in the corporation by policy or law. Therefore there is little an employer can do about them. But CME leave, CME expenses, Vacation etc. is negotiable and should always be negotiated.

Following list of benefits may not be complete but covers most of them. Many corporate employers also offer additional benefits such as day care, even pet day care etc.

HEALTH BENEFITS: Most of the employers offer health benefits. It is very important to have health insurance. Medical Bills are one of the most common causes of bankruptcy in the United States. A single catastrophic medical emergency can wipe away all your savings and put you under more debt.

Read your physician employment contract very carefully. It should say whether the employee or the whole family is covered under the health insurance. If your family is not covered then you will have to pay additional out of your pocket cost to get coverage for them. And you should if needed.

High deductible insurance has nowadays become very popular amongst employers. It requires them to pay lower premiums. For employees it opens up another venue to add to their saving and get tax breaks via Health Savings Accounts. Check with your accountant. However because of its high deductible, it discourages normally healthy people to go for medical check ups. So review the health insurance policy carefully before you make a choice.

VACATION: Please make sure the number of "paid vacation" or "paid time off" is always listed on your physician employment contract. Also it should specify separately the number of sick days, maternity leave, paternity leave, CME leave etc. It should also be clear whether holidays are included in the number of days mentioned or does it mean business days only.

CME EXPENSES: To maintain your medical license you have to complete certain hours of accredited medical CME every year. The medical CME expenses, including travel expenses ,are usually reimbursed by the employer up to a certain amount. That amount should be disclosed to you and written in the physician employment contract or physician employment agreement. It is also negotiable.

MOVING EXPENSES: Most of the times physician employers will offer to reimburse your moving expenses. If they do not offer it, be sure to ask. It can help offset your cost of moving to a different city or town. Remember, you cannot claim moving expenses you did not incur. So save your bills.

LIFE INSURANCE: Many physician employers may provide life insurance. Review the policy carefully because most of the time it is for a very small amount, i.e. $50,000. Also it usually pays the employer as a beneficiary to cover their cost of losing an employee.

In that case it is useless for you and I would suggest purchasing a separate policy. Larger corporations may provide more meaningful life insurance coverage.

DISABILITY INSURANCE: Most practices offer disability insurance. Do clarify if it is 'short term' or 'long term' disability insurance. Short term disability insurance usually covers disability for one to three months only. During this period physician employee will receive disability pay which is a percentage of your income. Long term disability covers disability up to age 65 and is preferable. Combination of both will give you maximum protection.

401K: Most medical employers offer 401K plans. Many of them match your contributions up to 3% to 6% of your salary . So if you contribute to 401K (which you should) you will 'earn' that extra money just by saving for yourself. Also it will give you tax breaks. Hospitals and larger institutions may provide 403b or other kind of tax shelters. Always find out how long you have to be employed by the corporation before they will consider you vested, partly or fully, to claim the employers contribution to the account upon leaving. Check with your accountant.

MISCELLANEOUS: Many larger organizations such as hospitals may provide wide variety of unconventional benefits such as day care for children (and even for pets at times!), concierge services for physicians, further education etc. All of these, based on your needs, may add value to the compensation package. ■■■

CHAPTER 15
Should I Get My Physician Contract Reviewed?

Every single day we commit ourselves to a contract - it can be expressed or implied. When you drop your clothes to the dry cleaner, when you send in your car for repair, when you buy a cup of coffee there is a contract involved. Some are more obvioius - e.g. you get a cell phone and commit for a year or two of service. Till now, for most of the medical residents, contracts are no big deal. Ninety nine percent of the time you have not been cheated. And for the rest 1% if cheating did happen - it did not do much damage. But do not bring this mind set when you step into the world of business-- or the world of practical medicine where you treat patients and practice business.

Stakes are high and will increasingly be higher as you move away from your graduation date. Now the damage to your career because of a bad contract will amount to tens of thousands of dollars. And trust me, it feels like a punch in the stomach.

Should you get your physician employment contract reviewed?
The answer is yes! yes and yes! You may have found your dream physician job, but if they offer you a bad contract - do not take it. Those words on 20 pages of paper can make you life miserable. And a good physician employment contract will protect you from such misery (After all everything has a brighter side to it).

Who should you get your contract reviewed from? Find a good attorney, who deals in business and contract law. Make sure he has experience reviewing physician employment agreements. Good attorneys are expensive, but the amount at stake is also high. Sometimes paralegals, who have experience reviewing physician employment contracts may be able to do it for a cheaper price.

Location of the attorney is also important. Always try to get a lawyer from the state where the physician job is located. Most likely, law of the state where the physician employer is located, will apply to the contract. And law varies from state to state.

Where do you find such attorneys? Websites like www.findlaw.com or www.lawyers.com are good sites to search lawyers from. Also ask for references from friends and associates. Never take the recommendation from the employer himself (There is something called 'vested interest'). ■■■

CHAPTER 16
Contract Negotiations

Welcome to the world of business. For us physicians, negotiating seems to be trivial, too downgrading a process reserved only for self centered people, selfish enough to ask what they want.

WRONG! Negotiations are an acceptable part of corporate America. Remember you are no longer a resident who is supposed to learn and to work eighty hours on bare minimum compensation. Now you are physician businessman with a degree and training and you live in the mighty American capitalism. By practicing medicine we do serve humanity but remember we have medical school loans to pay, a family to support, kids to send to school and plan for the retirement.

Always practice good medicine, ethical medicine and competent medicine. But practicing good medicine does not mean that you settle for a lower compensation, less vacation or lesser benefits. If you do settle for less you are serving your employer, not humanity.

Job satisfaction comes from performing your work you like to do with utmost competence and receiving adequate compensation for the same. How would you feel if you settled for $10,000 less in salary and three weeks vacation while your physician colleague gets four weeks vacation and higher pay doing the same work?

TAKE HOME MESSAGE. Negotiations are acceptable in business including in the business of medicine. It is accepted that you will try to negotiate your physician employment contract. Nobody minds it. That is one of the reasons the initial physician employment contract offered by private medical practices have two weeks vacation, no CME reimbursement, lesser compensation etc.

WHO SHOULD NEGOTIATE?

Most medical residents or physicians shy away from negotiations during their physician job search and would want their lawyers to negotiate with the employer. But remember not all lawyers may negotiate for you. Most of the lawyers will review your physician employment contract and tell you about the potential pitfalls. Then it is up to you to bring it to the employer. If you want your lawyer to do the contract negotiations, make sure it is clear in the beginning, before you sign an attorney client relationship.

There is a trade off as to who should negotiate the physician job contract with the employer. If it is the attorney then the process is usually slow, out of your control and can be expensive. But it is professional work, saves you from the pain of negotiating and may benefit you especially if your negotiating skills are poor. On the other hand you can decide to negotiate yourself. It also can be worth the experience as well as effective, educating and free.

HOW TO NEGOTIATE YOUR OWN CONTRACT

You can negotiate with your employer. There should be no stigma attached to it. Here is one of the ways to do it:

STEP 1. Ask the prospective employer to send you the physician job contract. Do not start negotiating until you receive the contract.

STEP 2. Review the physician employment contract at least three to four times word to word yourself. Make a list of sentences or conditions that bother you.

STEP 3. Get the physician contract reviewed by the attorney. He will give you a list of conditions which you may need to address with the employer. Also discuss the list you made in step 2 with the attorney and add relevant topics to put up for discussion.

STEP 4. Call your employer and tell him that there are some concerns regarding the contract which you would like him to address. His response to you will be "This is a standard contract for everybody." But politely insist that you would like some changes in it and offer to email or fax him the list. The employer may want to discuss it right then and there, but if the list is too long, do let him know. It is a good idea to give them some time to think on it. The employer usually will also run it by his attorneys.

STEP 5. Neatly type up the requested changes in bullet points on a word processor. Do make reference to page number, section, sub-section and line number. Also add an excerpt of the sentence you want changed and the language of the new sentence. Make separate bullet points for asking increase in salary, vacation days, sick leave etc. Send this list to the employer.

STEP 6. Most likely you will receive a call back from the employer, who by that time would agree to some of the changes and will decline the others. Now it is your turn to think whether the declined changes are significant enough for you to refuse the offer. Tell the employer to give you a day to think and then call him back later regarding your decision.

Remember you will not get everything that you wanted. The principle of negotiation is to meet half way where both parties feel they won.

STEP 7. If you feel that there is something which definitely needs to be changed then inform the employer about the same. Be clear. Usually this is a gamble because if the employer really cannot give it up then most likely he will go for another candidate. But remember he has spent some amount of time and money trying to negotiate the contract with you. So it is not easy for him to back off too. He will try to either convince you to give it up or may try to work out an alternate solution. If nothing works then he may either give in or let you go. You can execute this step very well if you have an alternate physician job or plan in hand. In that case power balance tilts in your favor. The upper hand in a negotiation is of a person with a plan B.

STEP 8. You will receive an amended physician contract from the employer. Again carefully review the contract and make sure the agreed upon points have been added or amended in the contract. Have the amended physician job contract reviewed by your attorney again.

STEP 9. If the new contract and conditions are agreeable to you then go ahead and sign the physician contract to seal the deal. ■■■

CHAPTER 17
Getting Ready for Your First Physician Job

After your physician employment contract is signed there is still a lot to do so you can start the new physician job on time. Proactive approach from the physician employee is always appreciated. Many of the processes listed below take months and are necessary for a physician to start his new job.

1) **MEDICAL LICENSE:** Make sure your application is submitted to the state medical board for medical license on time. Also carefully watch their estimated processing time and call them if you have not received the medical license in that period. Most of the time the State Medical Boards are quite efficient in dealing with applications. But they get hit with large volume of applications especially around the spring and summer time when the rush is at its peak. That is because most physicians change jobs during that time and the medical residents are entering the workforce. If your medical license is not approved on time, you cannot start practicing medicine in that state. Processing times can be long and may involve an interview.

2) **CREDENTIALING:** If you are entering a physician job then thank your stars that you don't have to negotiate with the insurance companies about the rates. However you have to get credentialed with the insurance companies so they recognize you as a provider and pay for your services. Medical License is a requirement for

final approval on credentialing applications. Most of the insurance companies will accept and start processing your application but will not approve them until the medical license is added. So ask your physician employer to send you the credentialing packet which will be a heavy bundle of forms. Most of the time the employers will forward those to you right after you sign the contract. You may ask the secretaries at their office to fill the forms prior to sending it so you don't have to do much other than sign.

3) **MALPRACTICE INSURANCE:** Get ready to come under the microscope of malpractice insurance companies. In the likely scenario where the physician employer is providing the professional malpractice coverage they will forward you appropriate forms to sign. Then they will be submitted by the employer to the insurance company. Malpractice insurance is not finalized until your medical license is approved.

4) **HOSPITAL PRIVILEGES:** For those who will also work in a hospital need to get the hospital privileges application turned in. Without hospital privileges you cannot see a patient there at all. NO EXCEPTIONS!

5) **HOUSING:** Start arranging for a house to live in. DO NOT BUY A HOUSE OVER THE PHONE !!!! If you think no one has done that then you are wrong. I know a couple of doctors who bought a house over the phone and lost a lot of money by ending up in a bad deal. Your best bet is to rent a house or an apartment for about six to nine months. Later on, once you are sure you are going to stick to your job and the area, then look for buying a house. By that time you will know the area well and can make an informed decision.

6) **BOARD EXAM:** Enroll in the board exams for your specialty and get them over with while you are fresh out of the medical residency. As you move farther away from your graduation date, it becomes harder to find time to study for the medical boards.

7) **PROCEDURE CARDS:** Get you medical residency program to complete your procedure competency certificates after turning in your procedure cards. ■■■

CHAPTER 18

Are You Late for Physician Job hunt? Last Minute Strategies

Within the last three months of the medical residency, most of the residents should have landed a physician job. If not, but you are mulling over several physician job offers, then you are still good to go. But if you have not done a single interview yet or worse if you have not started applying yet, then you are really getting late. But do not despair, as there are plenty of physician jobs available. Those who have visa issues need to be extra careful about the deadlines for applying for one.

There are several strategies to catch up. These techniques can be used by the early birds too as they are very effective in getting the contract in hand.

1. NETWORKING: Talk to your attending physicians in the hospital and program. Many of them will be looking for a partner in the near future. May be you can fit into that role. Even if they are not looking, they may know someone, who is looking for physician employees.

2. MEDICAL STAFF OFFICE: Talk to the Medical Staff Office in your training hospital. They are usually aware of doctors looking for potential partners/ employees.

3. PICK UP THE PHONE!: Yes! pick up the phone and call up all the places you have sent your resume to. Ask them for the physician responsible for making hiring decision. Talk to the hiring MD and ask him if you can set up an interview to discuss the opportunity further. Many a times, a reverse interview offer like this does work.

4. PHYSICIAN RECRUITERS: Call the physician recruiters in your specialty and they will be glad to have you signed up somewhere. Why? Because that's how they make the big bucks.

5. FRIENDS AND SENIORS: Do not forget friends and seniors who are already employed or own their own medical practice. They can also hook you up with a physician job.

What if the worst fear comes true. What if you graduate and there is no physician job in sight for you. Well that is a rare thing and should not happen if you have read this book early enough. But even if it does happen, then you still have options of locum tenens and moonlighting. This option is not for you if you need a visa for employment. The biggest drawback of having a gap between residency and employment is that you will have to explain it on all your applications in the future. I hope this sets you on fire to get started! ■■■

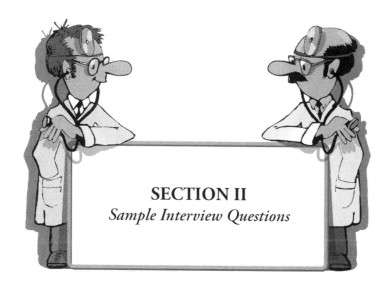

SECTION II
Sample Interview Questions

I am dividing this section into private and academia. But most of these questions are not exclusive. You may get a question from either section. But I want you to get an idea about different approach to interviewing. So consider reading both sets of questions as one complete sample interview.

There can be numerous right answers to any question. The correct answers may change with individual circumstances. But there are some ground rules to answer any question.

1. Always speak the truth. Lies will be caught, if not today then tomorrow.

2. If the truth may not sound good then say it in a positive way.

3. Keep your answers short and to the point.

4. Never badmouth your previous employer. ■■■

CHAPTER 19
Sample Questions: Private Practice Job Interview

Q: Why are you applying in this area?
The medical group wants to know whether you are willing to settle in the area or not. They may also be curious to find out if you know somebody around, who may have given you information about the group's financial or professional status. Or they may want to know which media is most effective in advertising their job opening. Possible answers can be:

"I am looking for someplace warm to settle down."

"Most of my family is around the area"

"I love skiing and would love to be in the snow"

Q: Why are you leaving your previous job?
Every body is curious why you were not happy in the last job. Or were you laid off. Now your previous employer may have been the devil's spokesman and you may have been doing everything right. But still hold that urge to let them know about that scoundrel. If you do criticize your previous job then you will project yourself as a problem employee. Possible answers can be:

"I am looking for a better opportunity."
"I always wanted to move to this area."

"They do not offer partnership. And someday I would like to become one."

Q: Is there anything derogatory in your records that we should know?

The biggest concern here is to avoid hiring someone with a blemished professional record. This creates a hurdle in credentialing the employee with insurance companies, obtaining hospital privileges or malpractice coverage. Do not lie. Let them know the truth, as it will save you from many problems later on. Malpractice lawsuits are a common place and unless you have done anything out of the ordinary, you have nothing to worry about. Just say it in a positive way.

"I have been involved in a malpractice suit. I have made extensive changes in my practice of medicine to minimize any chances of lawsuits. For I know that even with all good intentions one may still end up in a court."

Q: What do you think about our facility?

The employer is gauging your interest in becoming a part of his work force. This is an important factor in offering an employment contract and carrying out negotiations. Be prepared to answer this question in a positive way without showing desperation to get the job. Point out specific details that you appreciated.

"I am impressed by the professional growth of this practice in the past few years"

"I like the idea of offering patients a one stop shop for various kinds of diagnostics."

Q: When will you be available to start?

Schedules in medicine are planned well in advance. Staff shortages even for a short duration may mean additional burden on the existing physicians or the expensive alternative of hiring a locum physician.

The answer to this question will have the most influence on a decision to hire in private practice provided you have the required credentials and a decent personality.

"I am finishing my residency at the end of June. So I am planning to start mid July."

Q: What are your plans for the future?

Searching for a physician is an expensive preposition in terms of both money and time. Everyone wants a stable employee so keep those dreams of starting your own medical practice to yourself. If the group is offering partnership then show your interest in that.

"For next few years I want to get practical experience in the field. I definitely will be interested in partnership at some point."

"Currently I am looking for a stable job with strong potential for growth in the future."

Q: What procedures are you skillful in? Are you willing to learn a few more?

Most insurance companies pay ridiculously low payments for office visits. Procedures in medicine are paid reasonably well. So to keep the practice viable either the physician has to see a high volume of patients or be able to perform a variety of procedures. Generally a successful practice is a combination of both. If you are skillful in one or more procedures that may help the practice to grow then you will be in demand. Your willingness to learn more is a positive feature.

"Sure! I would like to expand my procedural skills if given an opportunity to do so."

Q: Would you be willing to pitch in during staffing shortages?

People get sick and flights get delayed. They all need somebody flexible enough to tide over these minor setbacks. Remember! A practice does not close and patients have to be seen. If a substitute cannot be found the employer has to shell out cash to hire a locum. If you say no then you are not a team player.

"We all have our good days and bad days. If a work needs to be done, I will pitch in."

Q: How soon can you give a commitment?

As I have said earlier private groups do not wait for the brightest. If they think you are good enough they would want to finalize the contract as soon as possible. After all they are eager to wrap up the search and get to their business. Answer this question carefully. Never be too eager to say yes or you may loose your edge during contract negotiations. Be polite, show your interest and let them know that you have few more opportunities to explore and once you are done you will let them know. If you are done interviewing and you know this may be the best position for you then ask them to give you few days to decide.

"I do have couple of interviews to end which I will complete by the end of next month. But I am very impressed by your practice and it will be certainly on the top of my list. I would be able to let you know by next month end."

"Your group has certainly captured my interest. I do have to think over a few things before I make a decision. But I can let you know in next few days."

Q: What salary are you expecting?

You may never get this question as most of the time the compensation is declared to you before you come to the interview. But if you come across this question, never give a number. You can say that you would try to find out what is standard compensation for the position in the area and go from there.

"I am looking for a compensation package which is at least average of what is normal in the area. I would have to do some research before I can answer this question."

Q: Do you have any questions?

Well if you don't, you are not serious. Examples of some questions are:

"What specialties are available in this area?"

"What is the payor mix?"

etc... ∎∎∎

CHAPTER 20
Sample Questions: Academic Medicine Job Interview

Q: Tell me about yourself?

Yes here it is again. A very common icebreaker can be used effectively to give a brief introduction and highlight your strong points. Think like a salesman and sell yourself. If you know a couple of new or additional clinical procedures let them know about it. People going for academics should talk about their research and teaching experience. But keep it brief. Present a clear picture of yourself without being lengthy and boring.

Q: Where do you see yourself five/ten/fifteen years from now?

You have heard it before. The answer they are looking for is that you will still be in academics. Don't tell them you will be going for fellowship somewhere.

Q: What area of research do you want to concentrate in?

Careful! The answer to this question needs extensive research. Do you have enough educational and research background to conduct that kind of research independently? Is there a potential for securing grants? Does the university have capability of accommodating such research activity? Will the research add to the already diminishing glory of the institution?

Q: Do you have plans to do further training?

Are we going to loose you once you get into the coveted training program? Just as in the private practice the academia also wants a stable employee. However in certain instances a desire to do part time training to enhance your credentials may actually work in your favor. For example doing a Masters in Public Health.

Q: Do you have current grants? Have you secured grants before?
Private practice generates your salary through your clinical activities. In academia if you don't have the ability to secure a grant your salary for the research part of your clock should come from somewhere else. This may not matter if you are applying for mainly a clinical track.

Q: What do you think of our city?
Well if you didn't like the place where the institution is, chances are you may find a place of your choice soon after getting the experience.

Q: What made you choose this institution?
Again research is the name of the game. Elicit positive points about the university and how they fit well to serve you towards your goal.

Q: Why should we choose you? What are your strengths?
Very few times in life someone will be patient enough to listen to you blowing your own trumpet. Do it with full enthusiasm. Don't be shy. After all you have to sell yourself. Mention all your strong points. For example: your research background, strong academic credentials, passion for teaching, team spirit etc. Prepare well for this answer test you may fumble when it comes.

Q: What are your weaknesses?
Never ever tell anyone your weak points. It is an admission of guilt and a sign of weakness. Transform strength into a weakness.

" *Well! Sometimes I focus too much on my work and forget to enjoy life!*"

" My friends tell me I work too hard"

"I cannot stop thinking about my patients at home".

Be inventive but be reasonable. ∎∎∎

CHAPTER 21
Sample Illegal Questions and How to Answer them

Federal law prohibits employers to discriminate against the employees on the bases of age, gender, marital status, sexual orientation, disabilities, national origin, color or religion. Any question asked to find out any of these details is illegal. Do not react angrily to these questions. Many times the employer may not realize that they are asking an illegal question. Or sometimes they become comfortable talking with you and lose their guard. Handle these questions politely but firmly. You may choose to answer or not to answer these questions. Or you may ask for the relevance of the question in relation to the job and answer their concerns directly. Following are the few examples.

Q: How old are you? When were you born? What is your age?
The employer has the right to know if you are above 18 year of age or not and nothing more than that. So you can assure him that you are more than 18 years of age without divulging your age.

Q: Do you have children? When are you planning to have children?
Unfortunately in medicine if you have children or are planning to have one soon limits your ability to work long hours. But most of the time this should not bother the employer unless he is planning to have you work your tail off. Family also limits your ability to

relocate. In an answer to this question can assure the interviewee that you would be able to dedicate sufficient (Of course! Not all of it) time to your job.

Q: Are you married?
This may actually be a benign question. Spouse has a say in making a decision such as employment. Many times the employers would invite the spouse to the interview. They would like the opportunity to convince your spouse about how great their part of the country is to live.

Q: What other non-professional clubs are you a member of?
It is a tricky question to find out your political beliefs, sexual orientation, national origin etc. But I have not come across anybody asking it in the medical profession. Again you can ask them about the relevance of the question. If they are trying to find out about your hobbies and extra curricular activities then you may decide to tell them about it. ■■■

NOTES

Made in the USA
San Bernardino, CA
22 March 2016